Table of Contents

Introduction 2
   Evolution of a Diet 4
   Adapting the Diet 6
   Ketogenic Diet 8
What is the ketogenic diet? 9
   How does the diet work? 10
      Who is the diet suitable for? 11
      What age range is the diet suitable for? 12
      What sort of food is eaten on the diet? 12
Classical diet 13
The Keto Diet's Surprising Effect on Epilepsy 20
   How Ketones Affect Seizures 23
   Does the keto diet help? 28
      How does it work? 29
   What It Entails 44
   A Word from Verywell 57
Conclusion 58

Introduction

The ketogenic diet is a way of treating patients with poorly controlled epilepsy. The diet – high in fats and low in carbs -- works by changing how the brain gets energy to function. Although not well understood, this diet has successfully reduced seizures in many patients.

There's no denying that the keto diet still reigns as one of the most popular—and highly researched—

diets out there right now. In fact, keto was one of the top 10 diets listed as part of Google's 2019 Year in Search report. And per Reddit's 2019 Year in Review, keto was the most-discussed diet trend of last year, plus the r/keto sub-Reddit was the number-two overall fitness/wellness community in 2019 and saw a 65 percent increase in subscribers from last year.

The ketogenic diet is a very low-carb, high-fat diet that shares many similarities with the Atkins and low-carb diets. It involves drastically reducing carbohydrate intake and replacing it with fat. This reduction in carbs puts your body into a metabolic state called ketosis. When this happens, your body becomes incredibly efficient at burning fat for energy. It also turns fat into ketones in the liver, which can supply energy for the brain.

Ketogenic diets can cause massive reductions in blood sugar and insulin levels. This, along with the increased ketones, has numerous health benefits

In this book, we explore the potential benefits of the keto diet for adults and children with epilepsy.

Evolution of a Diet

The shift from fasting to an actual diet was rooted in research, A test of a high-fat, low-carb regimen on epilepsy patients and observing a reduction in seizures that equaled that of fasting. A study in the Journal of the American Medical Association in 1925 reporting a significant improvement in seizure activity in 50 percent of patients adhering to the diet. Coined the "ketogenic diet," the regimen quickly became standard treatment for epileptic seizures. People with epilepsy and their caregivers were trained to follow a strict ratio of protein and carbohydrates to fats: 1 gram of protein per kilogram of body weight, 10 to 15 grams of carbohydrates per day, and the remaining calories in fat.

The diet fell out of favor as more effective antiseizure medications were introduced, but in the past few decades it has regained popularity as a treatment for children whose seizures fail to respond to medication. Over the years, new variations on the diet have emerged, including a modified Atkins diet, a medium-chain-triglycerides (MCT) version, and a low glycemic index diet. "These variations evolved to help patients adhere to a more liberal version of the diet.

Adapting the Diet

The classic ketogenic diet pioneered by Dr. Wilder is considered the gold standard for people with medication-resistant epilepsy because it produces the most ketones. It also demands the highest fat intake and is often the most difficult to follow due to the strict ratios required in planning and preparing meals. In the case of a patient had to follow a three-to-one ratio of fat to carbs and proteins. So, for example, if a meal included 12.8 grams of protein (less than three ounces of meat) and 7.9 grams of carbohydrates (one cup of string beans), it would also have to include 62.1 grams of fat (roughly equal to four and a half tablespoons of butter, cream, and coconut oil). Achieving these exact proportions requires meal preparers to weigh and measure food for every meal.

That's not the case with the modified Atkins diet. "It relies much more on keeping track of and not going over low daily carbohydrate allotments [no more than 10 grams of carbs]. People on the MCT diet get their fat from medium-chain-triglycerides, a type of fatty acid that occurs naturally in some oils, which is also available as a liquid called MCT oil. Those who follow the low glycemic index diet eat foods with higher fiber content that don't spike blood sugar. All variations, if properly followed, put the body into a state of ketosis, which seems to be the key factor in reducing seizures, The results can be dramatic.

Maintaining the diet was challenging for Mon, who says it took several months to get into a groove. "It involved a lot of planning and special ingredients, some of which we had never cooked with before." Luckily, getting Madeline to comply was relatively easy, says Mon, despite having to cut her fruit consumption to 10 raspberries a day.

Ketogenic Diet

The ketogenic diet is one treatment option for children or adults with epilepsy whose seizures are not controlled with AEDs. The diet may help to reduce the number or severity of seizures and may have other positive effects.

Foods included in the ketogenic dietUp to 70% of people with epilepsy could have their seizures controlled with anti-epileptic drugs (AEDs). For some people who continue to have seizures, the ketogenic diet may help. However, the diet is very specialised. It should be carried out with the care, supervision and guidance of trained medical specialists.

What is the ketogenic diet?
The ketogenic diet (KD) is a high fat, low carbohydrate, controlled protein

diet that has been used since the 1920s for the treatment of epilepsy. The diet is a medical treatment and is usually only considered when at least two suitable medications have been tried and not worked.

The ketogenic diet is an established treatment option for children with hard to control epilepsy. However, adults may also benefit from dietary treatments. Dietary treatments for epilepsy must only be followed with the support of an experienced epilepsy specialist and dietitian (food specialist).

How does the diet work?
Usually the body uses glucose (a form of sugar) from carbohydrates (found in foods like sugar, bread or pasta)

for its energy source. Chemicals called ketones are made when the body uses fat for energy (this is called 'ketosis'). With the ketogenic diet, the body mostly uses ketones instead of glucose for its energy source. Research has shown that a particular fatty acid, decanoic acid, may be involved in the way the diet works.

Who is the diet suitable for?

The diet may not work for everyone but is suitable for many different seizure types and epilepsy syndromes, including myoclonic astatic epilepsy, Dravet syndrome, infantile spasms (West syndrome), and those with tuberous sclerosis. If you or your child has feeding problems, or has a condition where a high fat diet would cause problems, the diet may not be suitable.

The ketogenic diet can be adapted to all ethnic diets, as well as for people who are allergic to dairy products. The dietitian will calculate the diet and try to include foods you or your child likes.

What age range is the diet suitable for?
The diet can be used in children and adults of any age, although detailed monitoring may be needed in infants.

What sort of food is eaten on the diet?
There are different forms of the ketogenic diet. The types of foods

eaten and the way each diet is calculated are slightly different, but each diet has shown effectiveness, in randomised controlled trials, in reducing seizures for some people.

Classical diet

In this diet most of the fat comes from cream, butter, oil and other naturally fatty foods. The classical diet includes very little carbohydrate and protein. Each meal includes a strictly measured ratio of fat to carbohydrate and protein.

Medium chain triglyceride (MCT) diet

MCTs are certain types of fat. This diet allows for more carbohydrates, so may offer more variety. It includes some fat from naturally fatty foods, as well as some fat from a supplement of MCT oil or emulsion. This can be mixed into food or milk and is only available on prescription.

Unlike the classical diet's strict ratio of fats to carbohydrate and protein, the MCT diet is calculated by the percentage of energy (calories) provided by these particular types of fat.

Similar dietary treatments for epilepsy

The following diets have more flexible approaches, which may suit older children or adults. They are still medical treatments, with potential side effects, and need to be approved by the person's neurologist. A ketogenic dietitian needs to individually set the diet for each person so that it is safe and nutritious.

Modified Atkins diet (MAD) and modified ketogenic diet

The Modified Atkins diet and modified ketogenic diet (sometimes called 'modified ketogenic therapy') use a high proportion of fats and a strict control of carbohydrates. These are often considered more flexible than the classical or MCT ketogenic diets, as more protein can be eaten, and approximate portion sizes may be used in place of weighed recipes.

Low glycaemic index treatment (LGIT)

This diet focuses on how carbohydrates affect the level of glucose in the blood (the glycaemic index), as well as the amount of carbohydrate eaten. Approximate portion sizes are used rather than food being weighed or measured.

Is this a healthy way to eat?

To make sure the diet is nutritionally balanced, an experienced dietitian works out exactly how much of which foods the person can eat each day. To help with this, people have individual recipes, are given support on how to plan meals, and are guided on which foods should be avoided. As the diet can be quite restrictive, the dietitian will recommend any vitamin and mineral supplements that are needed.

How is the diet monitored?

To check that the diet is producing ketones, ketone levels are checked using a blood test, or a urine analysis stick, which is dipped into a container of your or your child's urine. The blood test involves a small pin prick on the finger (similar to monitoring diabetes). You can decide with your doctor which method to use.

Are there any side effects of the diet?

Constipation is common, partly due to a lack of fiber. This can be easily treated. Hunger, vomiting and lack of energy are also common at the start of the treatment, but these may decrease with time and may be avoided with careful monitoring.

Many people report an increase in energy and feeling more alert once they are used to the diet.

Does the ketogenic diet work?

A clinical trial at Great Ormond Street Hospital in 2008, and other studies since then, showed that the diet significantly reduced the number of seizures in a proportion of children whose seizures did not respond well to AEDs. After three months, around 4 in 10 (38%) children who started the diet had the number of their seizures reduced by over half, and were able to reduce their medication. Although not all children had better seizure control, some had other benefits such as increased alertness, awareness and responsiveness.

Other trials have since shown similar results in children. High quality evidence for the effectiveness of dietary treatment for adults is increasing. Research studies are continuing to investigate how the different diets work, and why dietary treatments are effective for some people and not for others.

How can someone start the diet?

You can discuss the option of you or your child starting the diet with your GP or paediatrician/neurologist.

The Keto Diet's Surprising Effect on Epilepsy

The high-fat ketogenic diet can help stop seizures in hard-to-treat epilepsy. Doctors and dietitians explain how it works and how it is implemented.

Luella Klein had her first seizure at 13 months and was prescribed antiseizure medication. But by the time she was two and a half, the drugs had stopped working and she had developed new symptoms, including a severely imbalanced gait.

During a visit to the Columbia University Medical Center in New York City, Luella underwent a spinal tap to measure glucose levels in her cerebral spinal fluid. Based on the results, she was diagnosed with glucose transporter type 1 deficiency syndrome (Glut1 DS), a genetic metabolic disorder that occurs when glucose, a sugar in the blood, doesn't reach the brain in levels high enough to be used for fuel. That lack of fuel disrupts brain growth and function and can cause a variety of symptoms, including seizures, movement disorders, speech problems, and developmental delays.

A doctor recommended a lady should be put on the ketogenic diet, a high-fat, low-carbohydrate regimen that is standard care for Glut1 DS because it provides an alternate source of fuel fat for the glucose-starved brain.

Fats for Fuel
Normally, the body converts the carbohydrates in food into glucose, which then becomes fuel for all parts of the body, including the brain. On the ketogenic diet, which restricts carbs and loads up the fat, a different mechanism kicks in: The liver converts fat into fatty acids and ketone bodies, chemicals that can cross the blood-brain barrier and be used as fuel and may even be anticonvulsant ,when the body is

actively breaking down fat into ketone bodies, which is measured by a simple urine test, a person is said to be "in ketosis."

How Ketones Affect Seizures

For years, doctors have observed that epileptic seizures, which are triggered by abnormal electrical discharges in the brain, often diminish when patients fast. Researchers have linked this phenomenon to ketonemia, a condition induced by fasting that occurs when the body produces ketones as the brain shifts from using sugar, its preferred source of energy, to using fat. That metabolic shift seems to disrupt the abnormal discharges in the brain.

You are forcing the brain to use a different fuel, We don't know exactly how it works, but it's almost as though the brain can't figure out how to produce seizures using this new energy pathway.

Fried bacon slices
Until you're on the diet, you don't realize how many carbohydrates you eat, says a patient, whose daily carbohydrate maximum was initially capped at 20 grams. Within a month of being in ketosis, she went from 10 to 20 seizures a month to less than half of that. Today, still on medication, she has almost no seizures. Whenever she feels like

cheating. She says, she reminds herself that the diet is not a sacrifice. It's a change in lifestyle. Seeing the huge improvement in her health also helps to keep her on track, she says.

Ketogenic Caveats
These diets do not work for everyone and should not be undertaken lightly. It's not a natural diet, and we're not meant to eat this way unless it's medically necessary.

Fancy scrolled slice of butter
Some doctors will take a child off the diet if there's been no real benefit within six months. A child neurologist who specializes in

epilepsy, always cautions parents about the need for medical supervision, especially since most people with metabolic epilepsy, such as Glut 1 DS, will have to be on the diet for the rest of their lives.

No patient or caregiver should implement any version of the ketogenic diet by him or her, there may be serious interactions with commonly used seizure medications, and the side effects of the diet must also be monitored.

The side effects can be numerous and serious. The diet may cause constipation, acidosis [when the body produces more acid than the kidneys can remove, which can cause rapid breathing, confusion, going into shock, and even death], an increase in cholesterol, weight loss, kidney stones, poor growth, and bone fractures. "Children and adults on the diet need to be followed very closely." Epileptologists should collaborate with clinical dietitians trained in the use of high-fat diets who can screen for early signs of diet-related side effects.

Worth the Risks

Despite the risks, uncontrolled seizures, especially in young children, are reason enough for many parents and caregivers to embrace the diet. In most cases, parents, many of whom are well informed and have done their research, are demanding the diet. That parents are thinking out of the box is a good thing because over the course of a lifetime, the cumulative effect of seizures can impair health.

Does the keto diet help?
Under medical supervision, the keto diet may help control seizures.

According to a 2019 review, the keto diet appears to reduce or prevent seizures in children and adults with drug resistant or refractory epilepsy.

The Epilepsy Foundation recommends the diet as a potential treatment for refractory epilepsy. They report that more than half of children with refractory epilepsy who follow a ketogenic diet experience at least a 50% reduction in the number of seizures. Moreover, according to the same source, about 10–15% of these children stop experiencing seizures.

How does it work?

When a person is on the keto diet, their body does not receive enough carbohydrates to burn for energy, so it must use fat instead. Burning fat for fuel causes acids called ketones to build up in the body. When this occurs, the body is in ketosis. To achieve this, a person must adhere to the diet for a significant period.

Ketosis also occurs during periods of fasting. As a 2013 study notes, people have used fasting as a seizure treatment for centuries, and scientists documented the effects of this approach into the 1920s. Even so, experts are still unsure how, precisely, ketosis or the keto diet helps people with epilepsy.

Epilepsy is a metabolic disease, and one theory is that the keto diet works by altering a person's metabolism. Neurons, or hyperexcitable nerve cells, in the brain may contribute to the onset of seizures. The keto diet leads to metabolic changes in the blood and cerebrospinal fluid, and these changes, along with other factors, may decrease the excitability of neurons. This could have a stabilizing effect on seizures, according to experts.

The keto diet can take time to have an effect. In order to see the benefits, people should continue with it for at least 3 months after reaching ketosis.

It is very important that a healthcare professional monitors anyone using a keto diet for treatment. They can ensure that the diet is having safe effects and that the person's body is really going into ketosis.

Children and adults

Both children and adults with drug resistant epilepsy can benefit from a keto diet. It may be especially helpful for people with certain types of epilepsy, including:

Doose syndrome

Dravet syndrome

Glucose transporter type 1, or GLUT-1, deficiency

Infantile spasms

Rett syndrome

Tuberous sclerosis complex

The diet may also be effective for children with focal seizures.

Children

Children of any age can follow a keto diet. Under the strict supervision of a doctor, a formula only keto diet may help control seizures in infants. Parents and other caregivers should receive guidance on meal planning and cooking, and they should be aware of potential adverse reactions to the diet.

Adolescents and adults

Doctors often do not recommend the classic keto diet to adolescents and adults because it can be difficult to maintain. They may instead recommend a modified keto diet that is more palatable and convenient. Experts suggest that around 30–40% of adults with epilepsy who follow a keto diet experience at least a 50% reduction in seizures.

However, fewer than 10% of these adults achieve a 90% reduction in seizures or stop experiencing them.

Risks and other benefits

Anyone intending to use the keto diet to control epilepsy should be aware of the risks and possible additional benefits.

Other benefits

A modified keto diet may provide benefits beyond epilepsy management. Adults on the diet may experience improvements in:

Alertness

Concentration

Psychological function

The quality of life

Risks

Children and adults who follow keto diets must see their doctor or dietitian at least every 3 months. These regular visits are important for monitoring progress and growth and checking for any adverse effects of the diet.

Risks of a keto diet include:

Constipation

Weight loss

Increased cholesterol or triglyceride levels

Irritability

Lethargy

Nausea

Vomiting

Kidney stones

Growth problems in children

Since the diet allows for few fruits, vegetables, grains, and other nutritious foods, supplementation with a carbohydrate-free multivitamin is essential. Once a person has maintained control over their seizures for some time, their doctor may suggest coming off the diet. Doctors usually recommend doing so after a period of 2 years.

It is important to come off the diet gradually, over a period of several months or longer. Suddenly stopping the diet can cause seizures to get worse.

Other diets for epilepsy

Some modified versions of the keto diet for epilepsy include:

The modified Atkins diet: This is also very low in carbohydrates and high in fat. It does, however, allow for a greater choice of foods. It is important to count carbohydrates and ensure that the body is receiving enough calories from fats.

The low-glycemic index diet: This diet also has a high fat allowance, but it permits more protein than the keto diet.

The medium-chain triglyceride (MCT) diet: This is similar to the classic keto diet, but each meal tends to include fat from MCTs, such as those in oils or emulsions. It allows more freedom when choosing carbohydrate and protein sources.

Epilepsy and foods

At present, there is no evidence that any type of food generally triggers epilepsy seizures. There is a rare type of epilepsy, called reflex epilepsy, in which certain foods can trigger seizures. These triggers vary from person to person.

Some people with epilepsy report that specific food additives can trigger seizures. Potential triggers include:

Artificial sweeteners

Food colorings

Monosodium glutamate or MSG

Preservatives

Epilepsy and beverages

Some drinks can contribute to seizures or affect epilepsy medications.

These beverages may contain:

Alcohol: Alcohol can trigger seizures in some people. Anyone who believes that this is a trigger should avoid it.

Caffeine: Some research indicates that caffeine increases the risk of seizures, but that continued use may protect against seizures in some cases. Caffeine may also make some medications for epilepsy less effective, especially topiramate.

Grapefruit juice and pomegranate juice: These may increase the risk of adverse reactions to some epilepsy medications, including carbamazepine, diazepam, and midazolam.

Anyone with concerns about how foods or drinks may be affecting their seizures or medications should speak to a doctor.

Why do doctors recommend this kind of diet for people with epilepsy?

The ketogenic diet can reduce the frequency of seizures. In clinical trials of people with treatment-resistant epilepsy meaning they've tried a number of antiepileptic medications and continued to experience seizures the ketogenic diet typically reduces the number of seizures by 50 percent or more in half of patients. The number of patients that will go on to become seizure-free after adopting a ketogenic diet is much smaller some studies say it's as low as 0 percent of patients and in others it's closer to 20 percent.

How does the diet reduce seizures?

During a seizure, networks of neurons fire when they are not supposed to. This can happen because the brain cells are more excitable and are releasing lots of excitatory neurotransmitters, like glutamate. Or it could be that neighboring brain cells aren't able to suppress the spread of excitability like they normally would using inhibitory neurotransmitters like gamma-aminobutyric acid, or GABA.

The ketogenic diet reduces the amount of glutamate in the brain and enhances the synthesis of GABA, making it less likely for a seizure to occur. The diet can also reduce inflammation in the brain, and inflammation due to infections like meningitis, encephalitis, or autoimmune disorders can trigger seizures.

There have also been a couple of really interesting studies recently that examined how the ketogenic diet can alter the gut microbiome, the trillions of microorganisms inhabiting the digestive tract. These studies found the ketogenic diet can increase certain bacteria species that promote an increased proportion of GABA to glutamate in the brain.

Why do you think lifestyle modifications like the ketogenic diet can be important for people with epilepsy?

For patients with treatment-resistant epilepsy, the dose of a drug or combination of drugs necessary to stop seizures can sometimes cause significant sedation. I've seen instances where patients have been able to control their seizures, but their quality of life is really impacted by side effects.

In talking with my patients, a major part of epilepsy they struggle with most is the lack of control. They worry about going out in public and suddenly having a seizure there's just no predictability to it whatsoever, and I think that causes major anxiety. A diet is something in their environment they can control. They can be in control of their treatment and seizures, and I think that empowers them.

What It Entails

The ketogenic diet for epilepsy is a very high-fat diet with just enough protein for body maintenance and growth, and very low amounts of carbohydrate. When fats are broken down for energy, the body goes into what's called a ketogenic state, in which the body generates molecules called ketones. The goal of the KDE is for the brain to use ketones for energy rather than glucose (sugar) as much as possible.

Ketones are (largely) water-soluble, so they are easily transported to the brain. The brain cannot use fatty acids for energy, but it can use ketones for a large portion of its energy requirements.

The KDE is usually begun in a hospital setting and often begins with a one- to two-day fasting period, though there may be a trend away from both of these requirements. After determining the proper amount of protein (depending on age, etc.), the diet is structured as a ratio of fat grams to protein grams, plus carb grams. It usually begins with a 4 to 1 ratio and can be fine-tuned from there. The diet is often calorie and fluid-limited.4? Additionally, no packaged low-carb foods (shakes, bars, etc.) are allowed for at least the first month.

Because a gram of fat has more than twice the calories of a gram of protein or carbohydrate, this equation means that at least 75% of the calories in the diet come from fat. This is a very strict diet, and it takes time to learn how to put together meals that fit the formula. All food must be weighed and recorded. Weaning off the diet is often attempted after two years, though some children are kept on it for longer.

ketogenic diet calorie distribution

Why It Works

Researchers are beginning to understand why the ketogenic diet works to lower seizure frequency. According to a 2017 review of studies, it appears that several mechanisms may be at work, including the following.

The diet appears to alter ketone metabolism in the brain in a way that enhances the brain's ability to produce the neurotransmitter GABA, which has a calming effect on the brain. The diet has significant anti-inflammatory and anti-oxidative impacts, which appear to alter the way some genes involved in epilepsy, are expressed.

Certain fatty acids featured in the diet have anticonvulsant effects and have even been shown to boost the effects of valproic acid—a common anti-seizure medication.

Polyunsaturated fatty acids in the diet may prevent brain cells from becoming overexcited.

Decanoic acid, which is part of the diet as well, appears to have a direct inhibitory reaction on the AMPA receptors in the brain. These receptors are believed to play a role in epilepsy and are the target of some epilepsy medications.

Effects on a key sensor of cellular energy appear to help prevent excessive firing of brain cells.

The diet may impact circadian activities and the expression of a growth factor in the brain in a beneficial way.

Effectiveness

Studies generally show that about a third of children with epilepsy who follow the ketogenic diet will have at least a 90% reduction in seizures, and another third will experience a reduction of between 50% and 90%. This is remarkable, considering that these patients are generally those whose seizures are not well-controlled with medications.

In Adults
A growing number of studies have been done on the KDE and modified Atkins Diet in adults with seizure disorders, and the results are similar to studies with children. One 2014 study reported that 45% of adolescent and adult participants saw a reduction of seizure frequency of 50% or greater. Tolerability

appeared better in those with symptomatic generalized epilepsy.

Interestingly, it was more difficult to keep adults on the diet, since they obviously have more control over what they eat. Research is still limited in this area and more trials are needed.

In Pregnancy
A 2017 report on use of these diets during pregnancy suggests they may be an effective way to control seizures and could possibly allow pregnant women to use lower doses of epilepsy medication. However, the

safety of this still needs to be examined.

Work With Your Medical Team
It is vital that anyone using this diet for a seizure disorder do it under the supervision of an experienced physician and dietitian. Many individual variations can influence the exact diet recommendations for each person, and coordinating this eating plan with medications can be tricky. It's not something you should ever attempt on your own.

A Typical Day's Menu
Below is a shortened description of a menu. It's meant to give the idea of what children eat on the diet, not

serve as an exact prescription. Remember, all of these foods are carefully weighed and measured.

Breakfast: Eggs made with heavy cream, cheese, and butter; small serving of strawberries, pineapple, or cantaloupe

Lunch: Hamburger patty topped with cheese; cooked broccoli, green beans, or carrots with melted butter; whipped heavy cream

Dinner: Grilled chicken breast with cheese and mayonnaise; cooked vegetables with butter; whipped heavy cream

Snacks: Whipped heavy cream, small servings of fruit, sugar-free gelatin

Variations substitute coconut oil or MCT oil for some of the heavy cream and butter.

Eating While at School

With a school-aged child, keeping them on the diet during the school day is difficult but essential. Thinking and planning ahead can help you be successful. You may want to try some of the following strategies:

Talk to your child: Make sure your child understands the diet and why sticking to it is essential. Let them know they shouldn't trade food with other kids. As hard as it is, they also shouldn't eat food from vending machines or treats handed out in class.

Talk to the school: The teacher, guidance counselor, nurse, and administration all need to be aware of your child's special dietary needs (as well as other health-related matters). You'll want to have regular conversations with them, and you may want to have a 504 plan or individualized education plan (IEP) in place as well.

Become a planner: Gather several recipes for appropriate meals that can make convenient, easy-to-pack lunches. If possible, you may want to provide appropriate treats for your child for holiday parties and other special events that you may know about ahead of time. The Charlie Foundation and Clara's Menu are good resources for child-friendly keto recipes.

Educate family members: It's important that family members and any regular caregivers know how to prepare a meal for the child with epilepsy.

Establish routines: The timing of meals and snacks needs to be consistent in order for your child's glucose levels to remain as stable as possible. You may need to work with your child's teacher(s) on this.

Involve a friend: Having a friend at school who understands the importance of your child's diet may help them feel less awkward about being "different" and give them someone to lean on for support when needed. Make sure your child is OK with this and give them input on which friend to choose.

You'll also want to make parents of your child's friends aware of the special diet and that what some people may consider "a little harmless cheating" may not be harmless at all. It's a good idea to provide food for your child to take to parties and playdates.

How to Raise Kids Who Are on a Special Diet

Alternatives to the Super-Strict Ketogenic Diet

The Modified Atkins Diet is a popular alternative that helps many who find the ketogenic diet too difficult to adhere to. This diet is far less restrictive, as calories, fluids, and proteins are not measured.

The diet begins with 10 grams of carbohydrate per day for the first month, which slowly increases to 15 or 20 grams. It is similar to the very strict induction phase of the standard Atkins diet.

Research suggests participant achieved better seizure control when on the KDE. A 2016 study agreed that this is the case for children under 2, but that the diets have similar outcomes for older children. It also noted that the modified Atkins diet has fewer serious side effects and better tolerability.

A Word from Verywell

Because a high-fat diet runs counter to general beliefs about healthy eating, you may face criticism for putting your child on it. These critics are generally well-meaning, but uninformed. In the end, it's up to you and your child's medical team to determine the best course of action when it comes to safeguarding your child's health.

If you have questions or concerns about how a ketogenic diet may affect your child, bring them up with your doctor. Before starting the KDE, be sure you understand all of its nuances and are able to stick with it as prescribed.

Conclusion

The keto diet may be an effective treatment for people with drug resistant epilepsy. While the diet can be suitable for people of any age, children and infants may experience the greatest benefits because they can stick to the diet most easily.

Adolescents and adults may do better on a modified version of the keto diet, such as the modified Atkins diet or the low-glycemic index diet. A healthcare provider should carefully monitor anyone using a keto diet as a treatment. This is especially crucial for children and particularly infants. A doctor and dietitian can observe a person's progress, recommend supplements, and check for adverse effects.

Made in the USA
Columbia, SC
28 December 2024